Chakras & Meridians

MICHIO KUSHI
With Edward Esko

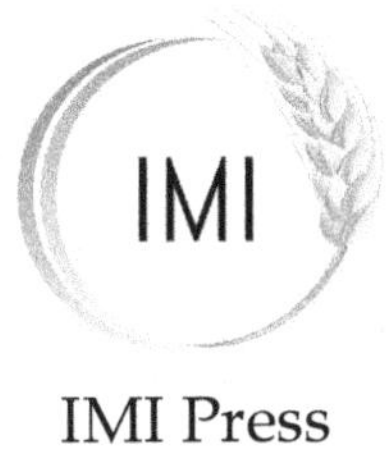

IMI Press

Chakras & Meridians

Contents

Chakras & Meridians
Copyright © 1993/2018 by Michio Kushi and Edward Esko
Calligraphy by Naomi Ichikawa

ISBN-13: 978-1986286046
ISBN-10: 1986286045

IMI Press
A Division of the International Macrobiotic Institute
P.O. Box 2051, Lenox, Mass. 01240
First Edition: April 2018
www.InternationalMacrobioticInstitute.com

INTRODUCTION

As Michio Kushi has pointed out in his lectures around the globe, in Japan life energy is called "Ki," in China, "Ch'i," and in India, "Prana." These terms are translated loosely as "life force." In Japan the character for Ki (shown below) is made up of two parts. The outer part depicts the universe endlessly streaming out from infinity. The inner part shows the image of a rice plant. When you see rice and other grains growing in the field, you may notice that they share a common characteristic. Tiny hair like structures project from each grain. These are called "awns." Merriam-Webster defines "awn" as: "One of the slender bristles that terminate the glumes of the spikelet in some cereal and other grasses." The awns point toward the universe; they point up toward heaven. Like tiny antenna, they conduct energy, or Ki, from the cosmos. When we eat grain as our main food, we are receiving energy directly from the universe. That is why eating grain was thought to be essential for developing higher consciousness. Spiritual traditions around the world emphasize eating grain as the main food. That concept is symbolized in the character for Ki.

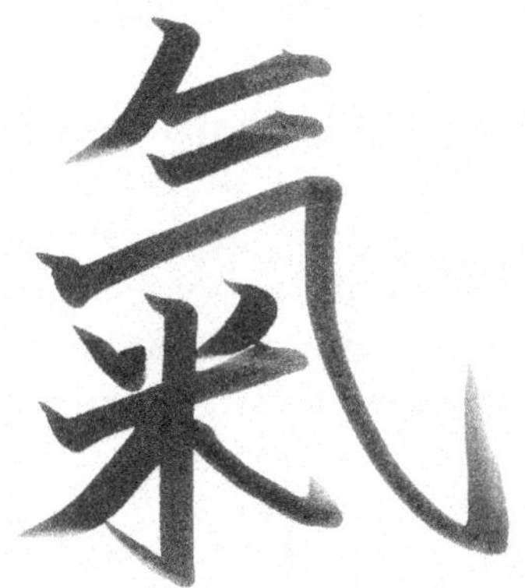

The Chinese character for Ki, or "life energy"

As Michio explains in this book, human life exists between two huge streams of energy. One stream, referred to as "heaven's force," is coming in from the universe, pressing on all sides toward the surface of the earth. Heaven's force enters the top of the head. It runs along a vertical channel deep within the body and animates all of our life functions. Heaven's force exits from the lower body. Meanwhile, because the earth is spinning, it gives off an opposite force. Earth's force emanates from the core of the planet and spirals outward. It is outbound, upward, and expanding. It produces diffusion, lightness, and dispersion. Earth's force enters the lower body and runs along the vertical channel in the opposite direction before exiting at the top of the head.

On earth, heaven's incoming energy enters most powerfully at the poles. Energy that enters at the North Pole collides deep within the earth with energy entering at the South Pole. A highly charged center arises there — the earth's core — comprised of molten metals such as iron. The highly charged core is spinning and giving off electromagnetic force that radiates outward, forming lines of energy at the surface. These highly charged lines give rise to mountain ranges. Earth's mountain ranges also exist deep below the ocean, for example, the mid-Atlantic and mid-Pacific ranges. Energy lines also exist in the form of the borderlines between the earth's tectonic plates. These areas are highly charged, so that when the earth's plates slip, a high-energy event known as an earthquake occurs.

We see a similar pattern in fruits and vegetables. In a pumpkin, energy enters at the top through the stem. It forms the central area known as the core. The core is hollow. Highly energized seeds form in this hollow core. Each seed contains the germ of the organism and can sprout and grow into a new plant. On the surface, we see ridges, which are the lines of energy that radiate from the central core. Lines or ridges are visible on cucumbers, squash, watermelon, and on other fruits and vegetables. The ridges are like mountain ranges. Energy comes in, creates the core, and radiates out toward the surface. The ridges are the plant's energy meridians.

Like the earth, the human body has a central core of energy. The central core is the vertical line that runs deep within the body, uniting the forces of heaven and earth. It is here that life energy is strongest.

We can live without a hand or an arm, but we cannot live without the functions, that arise along this central channel. It is here that seven highly charged energy centers, or *chakras*, arise. Energy from the chakras radiates outward. Some radiates up toward the surface of the body. This energy runs beneath the skin along clearly defined pathways. These energy lines are referred to as *meridians.*

There are twelve major meridians along which there are numerous highly charged points. As Michio has pointed out, the meridians are created in response to the highly charged energy coming in from the twelve constellations, or groups of stars, circling the equator. The meridians are receiving energy from this horizontal plane, and make balance with the vertical channel linking heaven and earth. Thus, when we study a map of chakras, meridians, and points, we are actually studying a map of the universe. The knowledge of Ki, or life energy, is the missing link in understanding our relationship to the environment.

If you walk along a country road, you will notice many types of vegetation, including different types of ferns. What is the pattern of the fern? The fern has one stem that divides into two; left and right or yin and yang. Each division divides into two, and each new division further divides, in a continual pattern of one dividing into two, two dividing into four, four into eight, etc. That pattern ends in the formation of individual cells. It is known as *fractal* division, and occurs throughout the human body. Meridians run just below the surface of the skin. Obeying the law of fractal division, branches come out from each meridian. These branches continually divide, becoming smaller and smaller. At the end of each microscopic branch is a tiny spiral. Each of these spirals is a living cell. A similar pattern occurs in the universe at large. There are giant streams of electromagnetic force, which extend across vast distances of outer space, in some cases more than a billion light years long. These energetic filaments are akin to the meridians that channel energy throughout the body.

Like the meridians, these channels continuously divide. And also like the meridians, at the conclusion of each subdivision is a highly charged spiral. From the point of view of the universe as a whole, these spirals are tiny, microscopic in scope. However, from our perspective, they are gigantic.

Each spiral is actually a galaxy, like our Milky Way. Galaxies form in in clusters. These clusters are like groups of cells in the body, including the specialized cells that make up the organs. Clusters of galaxies then group together to form what are known as super clusters. Some super clusters are over a billion light years long. They are akin to the body's meridian and organ systems, as well as to the larger grouping of organs into systems such as the digestive, respiratory, excretory, and nervous.

Michio describes the human energy form, comprised of chakras, meridians, meridian branches, and cells, as the Tree of Consciousness. The Tree of Consciousness originates within the universe itself. Our physical body is created in the opposite way, from the material substance of the earth. The body is composed of minerals, proteins, fats, water, and air arising from the world of elements found on earth. These elements continually replenish and enliven the body through food, drink, and breathing. The nutrients in food are distributed to the entire body through the circulatory system, which is also formed through fractal division. The large arteries that comprise the circulatory system continually branch into smaller and smaller vessels, at the end of which are microscopic capillaries that supply nutrients to the cells. The interface between the bloodstream, which is a fractal system, and the invisible energy form, also a fractal pattern, creates human life.

Fractal patterns are the organizing principle of the body and of nature as a whole. We see that reflected in the structure of the brain, the nervous system, the lungs and respiratory system, the heart and circulatory system, and in the liver, kidneys, pancreas, and other organs and body structures. The human body is composed of multiple fractal systems; visible and invisible, physical and energetic, functioning as an integrated unit.

The secret to health lies in maximizing the flow of energy through these visible and invisible channels. As Michio has pointed out, we can accomplish this through our diet and way of life. Whole grains, for example, contain strong life energy. Grains with the outer husk attached can live for centuries and sprout into a living plant. That is one reason why whole grains are an essential part of a healthy lifestyle.

By selecting food properly, we maximize life energy. Proper cooking is also essential. Cooking adds energy to food and accelerates the release of the energy and nutrients stored in foods. Cooking is a form of pre-digestion that helps break down plant fibers and release stored energy and nutrients. Foods such as whole grains and beans are hard and compact. We need to soften them in order to process them efficiently. Cooking is the first step in this process. As you will discover in this book, the guidelines and recommendations of the macrobiotic way of life are aimed at vitalizing Ki or life energy. These recommendations are presented from the perspective of life energy. In these pages you will gain an entirely new understanding of the importance of diet and daily life in creating health.

The material in this book is from lectures by Michio Kushi. It first appeared in the book *Holistic Health through Macrobiotics* published in 1993 by Japan Publications. It was in that book that the relation between the chakras and meridians, including the origin of the meridians, was first presented, together with the role of meridians as channels of consciousness. We have extracted that material for publication in this updated volume. IMI Press is grateful for having access to this timeless material and making it available to readers today and in the future.

Edward Esko
Former Director of Education, Kushi Institute (KI)
Founder, International Macrobiotic Institute (IMI)

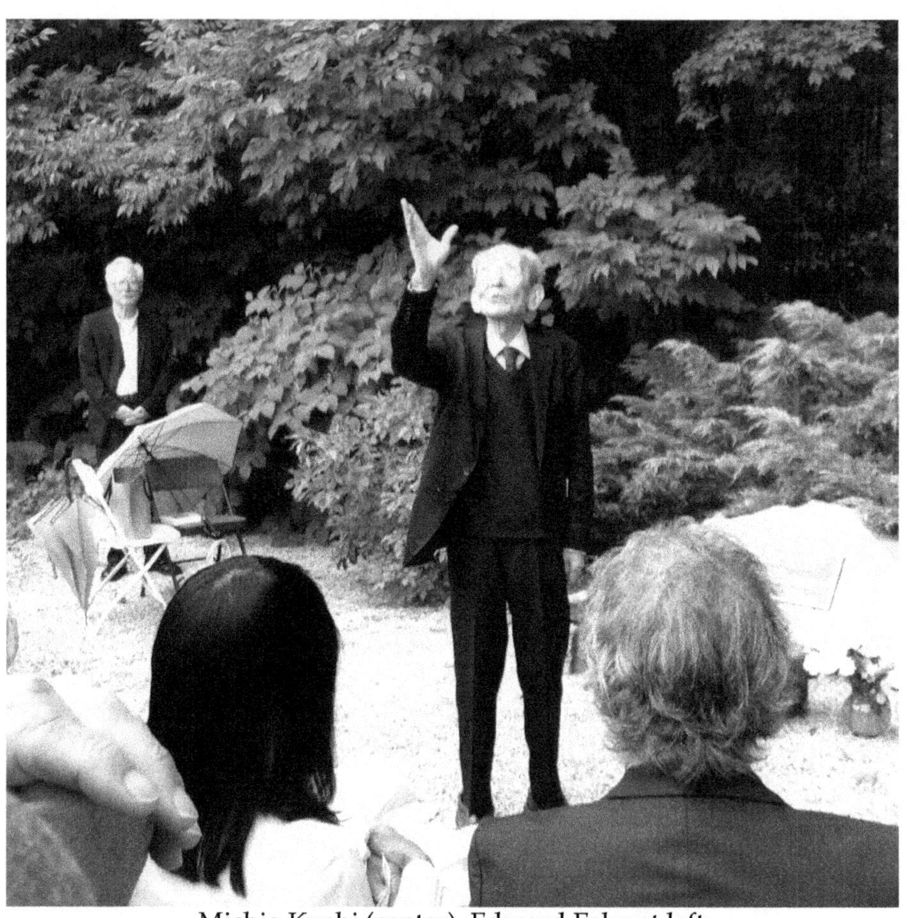

Michio Kushi (center). Edward Esko at left

THE WAY TO HEALTH

Spiritual awakening is the most important issue in health and healing. Self-reflection, leading to an awareness of the endless order of the universe, is the basis for healing the body, mind, and spirit. Self-reflection leads us to give up self-destructive habits and bring our way of eating and living into greater harmony with nature. A balanced, macrobiotic diet based on whole cereal grains, beans, fresh local vegetables, and other whole natural foods is the most basic reflection of a way of life in harmony with nature. A balanced diet provides the biological foundation for genuine health, while the spiritual foundation is provided by a deep sense of gratitude toward nature, the universe, and life itself.

A peaceful mind is fundamental to achieving good health. It is important for us to minimize stress and relax mentally and physically. Macrobiotic healing encourages everyone to have a peaceful mind and a positive attitude toward life. However, in today's society, when a person develops a chronic illness, he or she may receive a negative prognosis from his or her doctor. A negative prognosis has the opposite effect. It limits a person's freedom and causes stress and anxiety. It can have a negative effect on the outcome of an illness.

In order to overcome a negative prognosis, it is important for a person to create a positive vision for the future while at the same time taking constructive steps to change his or her current way of life. Making an optimistic plan for the future can be very helpful in this regard. The quality of our environment has a powerful effect on our health. A natural, non-toxic environment supports the process of healing, while an artificial, toxic environment limits it.

Concrete buildings, fluorescent lights, the artificial materials used in clothing and home furnishings, and the constant vibration of televisions, air conditioners, computers and other electronic devices, electric stoves, and microwave ovens disrupt the natural flow of healing energy. It is important to live as close to nature as possible. A regular daily life, in which we live in harmony with the cycle of day and night by being active during the day and getting adequate rest at night, enhances the recovery of health. Eating regular meals and keeping a reasonable daily schedule also helps to restore harmony in body and mind.

Our health depends on the active flow of blood and energy throughout the body. A daily half-hour walk helps activate circulation and is highly recommended. Other types of exercise are fine if they are enjoyable. However, it is not necessary to exercise to the point of exhaustion. If a person is unable to walk for an extended period, simply getting outside in the fresh air for ten minutes every day is helpful. In some cases, these measures are sufficient to restore health. In others, simple, natural home remedies may be necessary for a short time until balance is restored. These include internal and external preparations such as special dishes, drinks, and plasters made from daily foods. High quality home remedies are easy to prepare at home; they are inexpensive and non-toxic, yet highly effective.

Someone else cannot provide self-reflection and spiritual awakening. They result from our own self-realization and practice. We can learn from others how to balance daily food, make our environment and activity health supporting, prepare basic home remedies and give and receive simple energy treatments. Ideally, however, once we learn the basic principles of healthful living, we gain the ability to manage daily health practices on our own without having to depend on others. Macrobiotic healing thus encourages us to become more self-reliant and confident in managing our own health. The origin of sickness is our view of life. Therefore, macrobiotic healing begins with the central issues—spiritual awakening and self-realization, together with daily diet and activity—and employs peripheral symptomatic techniques only when necessary.

The macrobiotic approach is opposite to that of conventional medicine, which begins with symptomatic techniques while leaving these central issues completely untouched. It is for this reason that conventional medicine has been unable to stem the rise of degenerative disease.

Spiritual awakening is based on an awareness of our innate human freedom, including an understanding of how we create sickness and unhappiness through our thinking and behavior, and how we can change our condition toward genuine health. The purpose of macrobiotic healing is to guide everyone toward self-realization and the free management of their health and life. The central issues in health and healing—self-reflection and self-realization—are without cost, while the techniques employed by our current health care system are often very expensive. Ideally, health should be the result of daily life itself, including our way of thinking, diet, and activity. The way to health should be simple rather than complicated, affordable rather than expensive, and accessible to everyone. Moreover, the way to personal health should be the same as the way to social and planetary health. Creating a healthy and peaceful future for all people on earth is actually the goal of macrobiotic healing.

****

Once I was invited to meet a well-known spiritual teacher from India. He was more than eighty and had millions of followers throughout the world. As soon as we shook hands, I saw that he had a serious heart condition. The tip of his nose was bulbous and expanded; in Oriental diagnosis, a sign of an enlarged and weakened heart. I also noticed other signs that pointed to heart trouble and saw that his condition was caused by eating too much sugar. I said to him, "Every day, you are eating sugar and that has weakened your heart. For the sake of your health, please stop eating it." He replied, "I appreciate your advice, but consciousness, not the physical body, is my main concern." I replied, "Even if consciousness is our main concern, we still need to know how to take care of the body; otherwise, it is difficult to understand what consciousness is or how it functions." His disciples were surprised at my directness.

To this he answered, "I am taking care of people's consciousness and spirituality, I am not concerned with food." So finally I said, "Okay, fine, but anyway stop eating sugar." After bowing to each other, we parted. Several months later, I received word that he had suffered a heart attack and died. As a result, his worldwide organization fell apart.

This story illustrates the difficulty that people have in understanding unity between body, mind, and spirit. Many people believe that mind and body are separate, and that view has a profound influence on the way they approach health and healing. On one side are those who believe that the body is the most important factor in healing and that the mind is secondary. In the extreme, the body is thought of as a machine, with replaceable parts, and health and sickness are thought to result from exclusively physical causes.

According to this view, which is characteristic of modem allopathic medicine, the processes that govern healing are entirely biological or physical, and are not influenced by thoughts, emotions, or consciousness. On the other side are people who approach life from a metaphysical or mystical perspective. Like those with an exclusively materialistic view, people with a metaphysical view also see the mind and body as separate. They believe that the world of matter, which includes the body, is somehow less real or important than the world of mind or consciousness. Like the spiritual teacher from India, they believe spiritual progress is not influenced by physical health, and that faith, belief, or positive thinking is sufficient to overcome illness.

In reality, mind, body, and spirit are integral parts of human existence. It is impossible to separate them, and they are equally important in health and healing. The aim of macrobiotic healing is to establish physical, mental, and spiritual harmony in the person as a whole, and not just the relief of symptoms. It is, therefore, educational and seeks to deepen each person's awareness of the natural order that governs health and healing. It also seeks to equip each person with the understanding and practical tools necessary to take responsibility for his or her health.

Interest in the role of the mind in healing is becoming widespread today, largely as a result of the predominantly materialistic focus of modern, allopathic medicine. Accounts of faith healing (such as those reported at Lourdes), research into the placebo effect, and personal accounts describing the benefits of stress reduction, humor, and positive imaging in the recovery from illness have challenged the notion of mind-body separation.

That notion took root in the healing arts in the nineteenth century when allopathic doctors sought to establish scientific credibility by adopting the model of reality proposed by classical physics. In that view, based on a misunderstanding of Descartes's separation of mind and matter, the universe is a well-oiled machine that functions according to precise mechanical laws. Having set the vast cosmic machine in motion at some unknown time in the past, God was thought to be detached from the physical universe. There was little room for the human mind, or consciousness, in this grand, mechanical scheme. Consciousness was thus placed "outside" nature, as if it existed as a part of some separate realm.

As allopathic medicine adopted this "scientific" view, healing became less of a humanistic art and more of an impersonal science. It became less spiritual and more materialistic, less comprehensive and more specialized, less natural and more artificial, and less dependent on the body's self-healing abilities and more dependent on outside intervention. Along with the new idea of the "body machine" came the notion that sickness arose from purely physical causes. Since the mind was seen as invisible and intangible, its influence on the body — and on the process of healing — was deemed negligible. Moreover, according to this strictly materialistic framework, the mind or consciousness was thought to arise from the physical workings of the brain.

Consciousness was defined in purely materialistic terms; the mind was thought to exist only because the brain existed. The human spirit was thus confined by the closed, materialistic system of nineteenth-century physics. As this view took hold, medical science began an intensive search for the physical agents of disease. The role of the mind in determining each person's lifestyle and behavior — and thus his or her state of health — was considered less important than the role of physical agents such as bacteria or viruses.

These microscopic organisms were even considered to be more important than the condition of the person as a whole, which Claude Bernard, a leading nineteenth century dissenter from this view, referred to as an individual's biological "terrain." The role of the individual in health and healing was downplayed; people were disempowered and separated from their innate powers of healing. Health was no longer viewed as humanity's natural state, but regarded as being dependent on an individual's access to medical science and technology, thus setting in motion a cycle of co-dependency.

During the early part of the twentieth century, the theoretical model upon which this view was based began to collapse. New discoveries in the realm of physics paved the way for more comprehensive and dynamic paradigms of reality.

One such paradigm was the discovery that in the world of electrons, protons, and other subatomic particles, the consciousness of the observer not only influences but may also help create the phenomenon being observed. By reestablishing the link between consciousness and the physical universe, a link that lies at the heart of traditional cosmologies and healing systems throughout the world, this discovery revealed a major flaw in the classical worldview. Moreover, the discovery that thoughts and emotions play an important role in health and healing, a fact known by traditional healers for centuries, has revealed the limits of the model of health and disease based on the separation of mind and body.

Mental relaxation, a positive view of life, a strong will to live, and good human relations have all been shown to influence the healing process. On the other hand, negative emotions, such as anxiety, depression, and fear have been found to inhibit the immune system—and our self-healing ability. Positive emotions such as love, hope, and confidence have been found to enhance immune function.

Severe emotional or psychological stress has long been associated with increased susceptibility to illness. People who have recently experienced the death of a spouse or loved one often have higher than average incidences of cancer, arthritis, infection, and other conditions.

Strong feelings of grief can inhibit the immune system. In a study conducted by researchers in Australia, subjects who had recently lost a spouse were found to have diminished T-cell functioning. (T-cells are a type of lymphocyte, or white blood cell, and play an important role in the body's immune response.) In another study conducted at the Mount Sinai School of Medicine in New York, men who were married to women with advanced breast cancer were found to have a similar pattern of lymphocyte inhibition that lasted for several months following the death of their spouses. Their immune responses gradually returned to normal as their experience of bereavement eased. The heart and circulatory system also react to stress. Studies have shown that persons with repressed anger or hostility often have higher than average blood pressures and an increased incidence of coronary artery disease.

In one study of persons with blockage of the coronary arteries, those with the most severe blockage had the greatest degree of repressed anger and hostility. Persons with fewer repressed emotions had less severe disease. Those with severe arterial blockage angered easily, but tended not to express their feelings.

These characteristics are common among persons with so- called "Type A" behavior. Type A persons tend to be highly competitive, impatient, and constantly pressed for time. They are easy to anger, have trouble relaxing, and are prone to coronary disease. The opposite behavior pattern, labeled 'Type B," is characterized by a relaxed, patient, and even-tempered attitude with fewer feelings of time pressure. Persons with Type B behavior are also less prone to coronary disease.

The so-called "placebo response" is cited as an example of the power of the mind in overcoming the symptoms of disease. The Latin word *placebo* means, "I will please," and usually refers to an inactive substance that is given to a patient to satisfy the need for medication. When combined with the power of positive suggestion, placebos have been found to trigger biochemical changes in the body that aid the relief of symptoms.

Placebos have been used to relieve pain, induce mental alertness, and initiate recovery from the symptoms and signs of chronic diseases. When combined with negative suggestion, they have been found to cause negative side effects that are similar to those of powerful drugs.

Clearly, mind and body are not separate. They are the invisible and visible, back and front, and yin and yang of the one reality that makes up a human being.

THE MIND BODY CONNECTION

Investigators seeking to discover how the mind influences physical health have tended to focus on the biochemical pathways through which the brain influences various bodily functions. The positive expectations elicited by a placebo, for example, are thought to stimulate the cortex, which in turn activates the endocrine system, including the adrenal glands. The action of adrenal hormones in turn affects the body's organs and functions. Positive expectations may also activate the autonomic nervous system, and thus activate or inhibit various bodily functions. They may also stimulate the brain to secrete chemicals known as endorphins that have the effect of reducing the awareness of pain.

Thoughts, moods, and emotions also affect the brain's secretion of chemicals that carry messages between cells. These chemical messages are carried by neurohormones that travel through the bloodstream and by neurotransmitters that travel through the body-wide network of nerve cells. These chemicals are attracted to specialized receptors on the surface of body cells, and either stimulate or inhibit the activity of the cell.

The nervous system is not the only channel through which thoughts and emotions affect the body. Thoughts and emotions exist in the form of energy waves that travel through an invisible, body-wide network that connects each cell in the body. Until recently, modem medicine was not aware of this invisible energy system. This concept had not been encountered until investigators began to study the traditional healing systems of the East, where the body's invisible energy system was known and used for thousands of years.

This system, comprised of meridians, meridian branches, and chakras, may hold the key to understanding the interaction between mind and body. After all, human consciousness is an invisible, energetic phenomenon. Trying to understand it in terms of the biochemical effects it produces is like trying to understand what someone is like by examining footprints in the sand. In order to create a truly holistic paradigm, we need to embrace and understand the traditional concept of energy. The body's energy system represents the new frontier of health and healing. It holds the key to unifying mind and body, spirit and matter, consciousness and health.

****

The medical systems of India, China, Japan, and other Asian countries are based on the understanding and use of life energy. They go back thousands of years, and are derived from an ancient cosmology, or worldview, that saw all things in nature as manifestations of energy, or vibration. Ayurveda, the ancient medicine of India, which dates back at least 5,000 years, taught that all things in the universe — from the tiniest atom to the largest galaxy — are different forms of universal consciousness or energy.

In Japan and China, an invisible force, referred to as *Ki,* or *Ch'i,* was thought to permeate the universe. According to the centuries-old philosophy of Oriental medicine, Ki, or life energy, manifests in countless material and nonmaterial forms, including mind and body, heaven and earth, spirit and matter. When it takes more inert, condensed forms, it appears as matter, and when it assumes more diffused, dynamic forms, it appears as mind, consciousness, and other nonmaterial phenomena. The concept of life energy is basic to traditional concepts of health and healing. In Japan, for example, sickness is described as *Byo-Ki,* or "suffering Ki," meaning that illness is a manifestation of energy imbalance. In contrast the Japanese word for health, *Gen-Ki,* means "original Ki." It implies that health is our original natural state of being. Kahuna medicine, the native healing tradition of Hawaii, is founded on the same idea.

The Kahuna word for good health means "abundance of energy." Poor health is conceived of either as a weakness, or lack of energy, or as tension or blockage in the flow of energy throughout the body. The word for "healing" means to restore energy and achieve a condition of harmony or fullness.

The traditional concept of energy is not incompatible with modem science. New discoveries in the realm of physics have made it possible to unite scientific understanding with this ancient view. In the view of nineteenth-century physics, atoms were tiny, material points and were the final, irreducible unit of matter. However, when scientists began to subdivide and analyze atoms, they discovered that atoms are composed largely of empty space within which much smaller units known as electrons, protons, and neutrons are in constant motion. (Today, over two hundred of these subatomic particles have been identified.)

Moreover, when these smaller units were studied closely, it was discovered that they were not particles, but condensed packets of energy that had the characteristics of both intangible waves and tangible particles. They were material in the sense that they left behind tracks that could be detected with the senses, and at the same time were fleeting, impermanent, and nonmaterial. Thus, according to modem physics, matter is essentially composed of energy, or non-matter. That conclusion was reached thousands of years ago and articulated in the concept of Ki, or life energy.

Our planet is constantly bathed in cosmic energy. From the infinite periphery of space, energy is spiraling in toward the earth in the form of solar and stellar radiation, cosmic rays, and solar and galactic wind, together with light and energy from a countless number of stars, planets, galaxies, and other celestial bodies. Because this stream of energy originates in the cosmos, we can refer to it as heaven's force. Heaven's force moves from the infinite periphery of space toward the infinitesimally tiny point known as the earth, and exerts a condensing or contracting effect on the earth and everything on it. Because of its rotation, the earth generates tremendous energy. Heaven's force pushes everything down toward the surface of the planet.

Earth's force is the opposite: it spirals up from the surface of the planet and out toward infinite space. Together these forces charge the planet and everything on it. They are the primary sources of the life energy that charges all beings, and that animates every aspect of our lives, including the movements of our body, mental and emotional responses, and spiritual qualities.

In macrobiotics we borrow from the Chinese terminology to describe these primal forces. Yang—centripetal downward, and contracting—describes heaven's incoming energy. Yin—centrifugal, upward, and expanding—describes earth's outgoing force. Yin and yang make it possible to develop a classification of all phenomena, not only those on our planet but throughout the universe, into two complementary and antagonistic categories. Yin and yang reveal the interdependence and interconnectedness of all things. They unite the endless diversity of things into a simple and practical, yet comprehensive understanding of reality. And, because yin and yang describe the everlasting law of change, they make it possible to understand the past, predict future changes, and foresee the outcome of events, including the origin, present status, and future outcome of sickness.

Body, mind, and spirit are the product of these primary forces. Human life exists at the balancing point between heaven and earth. We are created by the fusion of these two huge streams of energy. In the body, they create two complementary "trees" that animate all aspects of life. One, which we can refer to as the Tree of Consciousness, is primarily the product of heaven's force. It is comprised of invisible energy and originates in the universe. The other, which we refer to as the Tree of the Body, consists of the physical, material body, including organs, tissues, and cells. The physical body is formed out of the material substance of the earth, including food, water, and air.

We exist at the intersection of heaven and earth, celestial and terrestrial, incoming energy and outgoing force. Achieving balance and harmony between the two primal forces is the secret of health, longevity, and day-to-day happiness. Achieving that harmony is the goal of macrobiotic healing, both on the personal and planetary level.

CHAKRAS & MERIDIANS

Heaven's energy spirals in toward the surface of the planet and enters the human body through the spiral, or cowlick, on top of the head. From here, energy streams downward along an invisible line running deep within the body. This primary energy channel charges the entire body and all its functions. It extends from the top of the head to the sexual organs. Heaven's downward force enters the top of the head, flows through the body, and exits in the region of the sexual organs. Meanwhile, an invisible stream of earth's force moves along the primary channel in the opposite direction, entering in the region of the sexual organs and exiting through the hair spiral.

The flow of heaven's and earth's forces through the primary channel gives rise to seven highly charged energy centers, which in ancient India were named *chakras*, or *wheels*. The chakras concentrate energy from the surrounding environment and distribute it throughout the body. The *crown*, or *seventh chakra* is located at the top of the head in the region of the hair spiral. Because of its position, the crown chakra is highly charged with cosmic energy and supplies this energy to the cerebral cortex, providing the basis for the images, consciousness, and sensations that arise there. Energy from this chakra radiates a gold color.

The next energy center is located deep within the brain, in the area of the midbrain. This focal point of energy is known as the *sixth,* or *midbrain chakra.* Energy is distributed from this chakra to the millions of cells in the brain. Brain cells function as highly communicative instruments, processing vibrations in a manner similar to a cellular phone, receiving energy from the cellular tower and producing images, sensations, and consciousness. Thoughts and images take the form of invisible, vibrational holograms projected onto three-dimensional space. Energy in the midbrain chakra radiates a silver-yellow color.

Heaven's force moves downward through the body and causes the uvula to develop at the back of the throat. It also causes a pair of glands, the adenoids, to develop in the form of spirals on either side of the uvula. Heaven's force also creates and activates the salivary glands, generating the production of highly charged liquid, saliva. Meanwhile, earth's force—which streams upward from the lower body—creates and charges the tongue, along with a pair of glands in the throat known as the tonsils.

As it concentrates in the throat, heaven's force produces another highly charged energy center known as the *fifth,* or *throat chakra.* The concentration of energy here activates the motion of the tongue and vocal cords, producing the human voice. It also stimulates the thyroid and parathyroid glands to secrete hormones. Energy in the throat chakra radiates a yellow color.

The *fourth,* or *heart chakra* is located in the center of the chest in the region over the heart. Here, the active rhythm of heaven and earth's forces produces the heartbeat. Contracting of the heart is produced by heaven's force and expansion, by earth's force. The rhythmic movement of the lungs is also regulated by the energy in this chakra, and energy from this center charges the heart and circulation, blood and body fluids, and the function of breathing. Feelings and emotions, including those of love, compassion, and sympathy, are produced here. Heart chakra energy radiates a pink color.

The *third,* or *stomach chakra* is located in the center of the solar plexus, about two inches below the base of the sternum. It activates the movement of the stomach and digestive organs and supplies the liver, spleen, gallbladder, pancreas, and kidneys with energy.

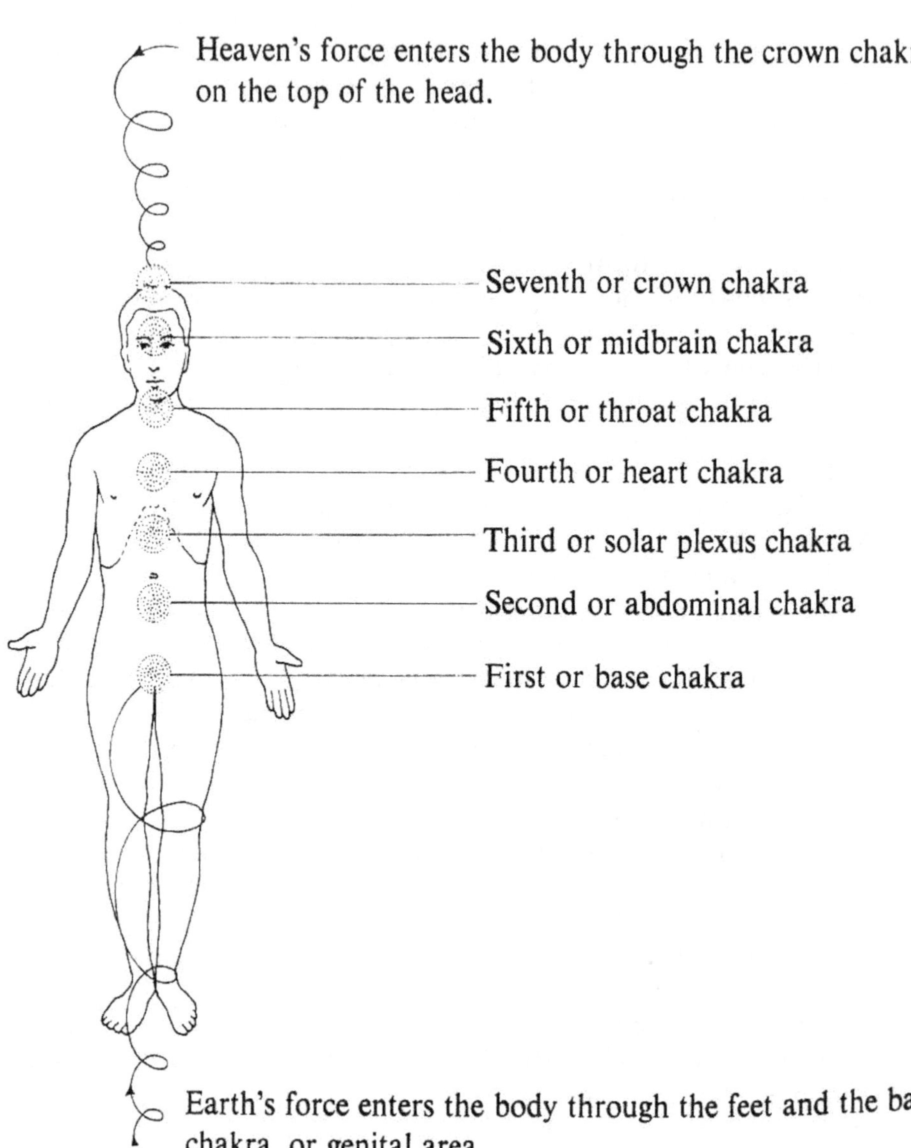

The seven chakras or energy centers

The stomach chakra translates the images and feelings generated in the upper chakras into the movements of the lower body, and activates the secretion of hormones and digestive juices. Energy in the stomach chakra radiates an orange color.

The *second,* or *hara chakra,* is located in the lower part of the small intestine, about two fingers below the navel, and is the central focus of energy in the lower abdomen. It is also referred to as *Ki-Kai,* or "ocean of electromagnetic energy," and *Tanden,* or the "central field" of energy. From here energy is distributed in waves, causing rhythmic expansion and contraction of the small and large intestines. Intestinal digestion, decomposition and absorption of food molecules and movement of the intestines occur because of the energy flowing from this chakra. Hara chakra energy radiates a red color.

In women, the hara chakra is located in the upper part of the uterus. It is here that implantation of the fertilized ovum takes place. The intense charge of life energy in this region stimulates development of the placenta and embryo, and after nine months, activates the contractions that occur during labor. Labor begins when the charge of heaven and earth's forces intensifies in the hara region, causing the uterus to begin rhythmic contractions. These movements begin in the hara chakra and spread downward in the form of a wave.

The *first,* or *base chakra* is located at the base of the spine. It charges the bladder, rectum, and reproductive organs, and activates physical and sexual vitality. Heaven's downward force exits the body through this chakra, while earth's expanding force enters the body in this region. Energy in the sexual chakra radiates in a dark red color.

The primary channel and chakras comprise the trunk of the Tree of Consciousness. The two chakras in the head form the roots of this upside-down tree. Although the central line conducts both heaven's and earth's forces, its primary energy source flows downward from the sky to the earth. On the earth, heaven's descending force is generally seven times stronger than the upward, centrifugal force generated by the rotation of the planet. Therefore, we can say that the soil that nourishes the Tree of Consciousness is the universe itself.

****

Like the trunk of a tree, the primary channel differentiates into branches. Each branch carries energy from the primary channel to the rest of the body. These branches are known in Oriental medicine as *meridians*. The Japanese refer to them as *Kei-Raku*, or "channels." Meridians radiate outward from the primary channel in the way that the ridges of a pumpkin branch outward from its central core. Although they are usually thought of as energy "lines," each meridian is actually a spiral, with the most peripheral orbit running near the surface of the body below the skin. Each meridian-spiral coils inward so that the central orbits are located deep within the body. Here, each stream of energy differentiates into numerous smaller branches that end in billions of cells in a process known as *fractal* division. Fractal division occurs in seven stages, with each branch subdividing into smaller and smaller units. Like stars that cluster into constellations, cells cluster into groups that are nourished by a particular meridian. These condensed cell clusters are the internal organs. The cells of the skin, muscles, bones, brain and nervous system, and glands also differentiate from the meridians and chakras and are part of this complex energy network.

The process through which the primary channel differentiates into meridians, meridian branches, and a cell is similar to the process through which the trunk of a tree differentiates into numerous branches and leaves, again, through a pattern of fractal division. Just as each leaf receives nourishment from the roots of the tree, each cell is constantly supplied with energy from primary channel and chakras. Cosmic energy is constantly streaming into the body, charging each cell and animating all of its functions.

Each meridian also has numerous direct channels to the outside. These channels take the form of tiny "holes" at the surface of the body. Energy from the outside enters the body through these holes, and is absorbed and incorporated into the general flow of energy along the meridian. At the same time, energy produced inside the body flows outward through these holes. Each hole is like a miniature volcano that releases energy. The body-wide network of energy holes comprises the system of "points" used in acupuncture, shiatsu massage, and other traditional Oriental therapies.

Although they develop through a similar process of fractal division, trees and human beings actually have an opposite structure. The roots of the tree are in the earth. Energy and nutrients from the soil stream upward through the trunk, and out through the branches to each leaf and flower. The tree's reproductive functions are carried on in the upper, most peripheral regions of the tree where flowers and seeds are produced. The roots of the human body are in the head, through which energy from the universe flows downward along the primary channel, charging the chakras, meridians, and cells. Unlike leaves that develop externally, cells appear deep inside the body. Our reproductive functions, which are similar to the fruit, flowers, and seeds of the tree, are not located in an upward position, but downward at the lower end of the primary channel. The human ovum is not fertilized externally, as seeds are, but internally. It develops deep within the mother's body rather than separate from the mother in the outside environment.

The uppermost chakras are the first to receive the incoming flow of celestial force. Thoughts and images produced in these chakras generate energy waves that travel down the primary channel, through the chakras, and out to the meridians. Consciousness waves then disperse through the minute network of meridian branches, arriving ultimately at the cells, in a process that is similar to the transmission of nerve impulses from the brain through the finely differentiated network of peripheral nerves. The nature of these consciousness waves has a direct influence on the functioning of the cell. Each cell is influenced by the thoughts, images, and vibrations produced in the uppermost chakras.

A calm, clear, and tranquil mind allows energy to stream freely through the primary channel and chakras. Bright, happy, or positive thoughts stimulate the flow of life energy reaching the cells. Dark, negative, or depressing thoughts weaken or interfere with the smooth flow of energy along these pathways, and diminish the supply of energy reaching the cells. And as we have seen, thoughts also affect the way brain cells secrete chemical messengers, and these also affect the body's cells. The speed at which consciousness waves travel through the chakras, meridians, and meridian branches is more rapid than the speed at which impulses travel through the nervous system. As a consequence, thoughts, images, and vibrations arising in the brain influence the cells through the invisible energy network before they activate the biochemical pathways described above.

The body and mind are one. Through pathways both visible and invisible, thoughts and images exert a profound influence on our health and well-being.

****

The chakra system is one of the keys to understanding the relationship between body, mind, and spirit. We are constantly receiving vibrations from our environment, both near and far. These include the full range of sensory inputs and more subtle vibrations, including those of consciousness and thinking. They travel from the periphery of the body to the brain via the nervous system. Images, thoughts, and emotions arise in response, and produce impulses that flow down the primary chakra line, charging and activating certain chakras. Depending on the type of energy that is produced, the chakras are either activated or inhibited.

The invisible energy system grows downward in a manner that is opposite to trees in the vegetable kingdom. The uppermost chakras become active early in life. They function in concert with the brain in coordinating our mechanical and sensory activities. The third, or throat chakra, becomes active soon afterward, stimulating the ability of speech and self-expression. Then, the energetic functions of the fourth, or heart chakra become active, and emotions and feelings, including those of love and tenderness, appear.

Intellectual ability develops next, and this capacity is centered in the fourth, or stomach chakra in the solar plexus. As the sixth, or hara chakra becomes active, social awareness begins developing. The seventh, or sexual chakra becomes active at about the age of fourteen for girls and sixteen for boys. Sexual and reproductive abilities are the last to develop and are an extension of the capacities centered in the hara chakra. Sexuality represents the condensed essence of all social relationships.

The chakras are centers for these mental and emotional capacities. The direction in which they develop—downward from heaven to earth—is opposite to the direction in which consciousness develops. Consciousness expands upward and outward, beginning with mechanical responses to the environment, followed by sensory awareness, emotional and intellectual responses, social and philosophical concerns, and ultimately all-embracing universal consciousness.

This process occurs in the form of an expanding spiral that counterbalances the contracting spiral through which human life takes form. As our consciousness develops, we are able to embrace larger and larger dimensions of time and space.

The meridians begin and end in the chakras. Each one is a channel for the vibrations of consciousness produced in the chakras. The body's cells are connected to the meridians through the meridian branches, and act as thought or consciousness centers. The meridians also channel energy from the environment and either activate or sedate the mental and emotional functions centered in the chakras. Mind and body are one, unified by the body's invisible energy grid.

THE LUNG MERIDIAN

The lung meridian begins at the stomach chakra and descends to connect with its partner organ, the large intestine. It then reverses direction, passes through the lungs, ascends to the throat, and moves out to the shoulder. From there, it runs down the inner arm to the outer corner of the thumbnail. Several inches above the wrist, a branch of the lung meridian descends directly to the index finger, where the large intestine meridian begins.

The lung meridian flows outward from the body and is charged with the earth's yin energy. The intellectual capacities generated in the stomach chakra flow out along the lung meridian in the form of waves. We can say that the lung meridian is a channel for the waves of the intellect. The strong current of earth's expanding energy that charges the lung meridian causes the intellect to become active rather than dormant. The meridian on the right side of the body (and the right lung) is powerfully charged with earth's force, and strongly activates the intellect. The meridian on the left side of the body (and the left lung) is strongly charged with heaven's force, and has a weak activating effect on intellectuality.

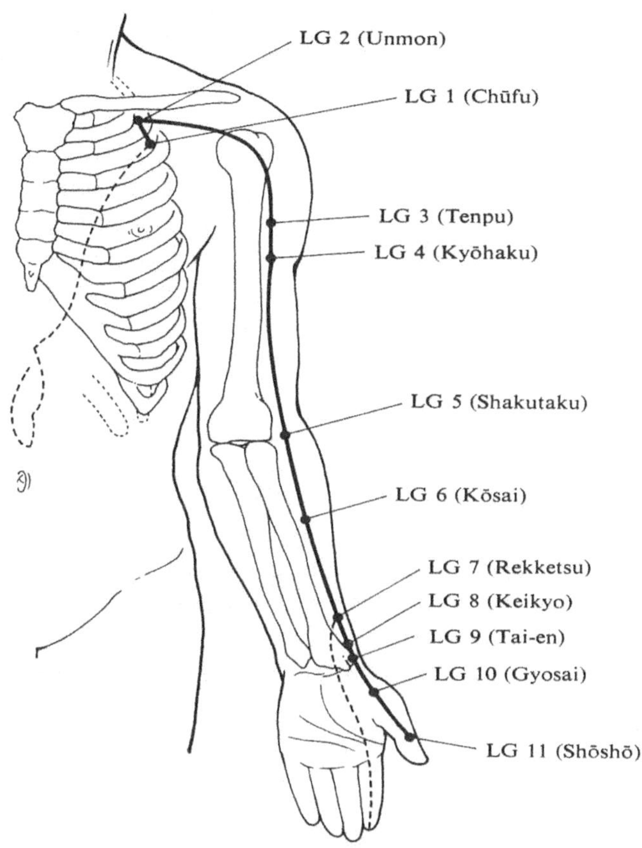

The lung meridian

THE LARGE INTESTINE MERIDIAN

The large intestine meridian begins at the thumb-side comer of the index finger and runs up the finger, hand, and thumb-side of the arm to the top of the shoulder. From there, one branch enters the body and descends to the large intestine and hara chakra. Another branch goes from the shoulder up the side of the neck to the face, crosses between the mouth and the nose, and ends at the outside comer of the nostril. At the end of the nostril, this branch connects to the stomach meridian.

The large intestine meridian receives energy from the hara chakra, and is a channel for our social awareness. On the whole, the large intestine meridian is charged with heaven's yang force, and thus has a stabilizing, rather than an activating, effect on social development. The meridian on the right arm has a weak stabilizing effect, as does the ascending colon, while the meridian on the left arm has a more powerful stabilizing effect, as does the descending colon.

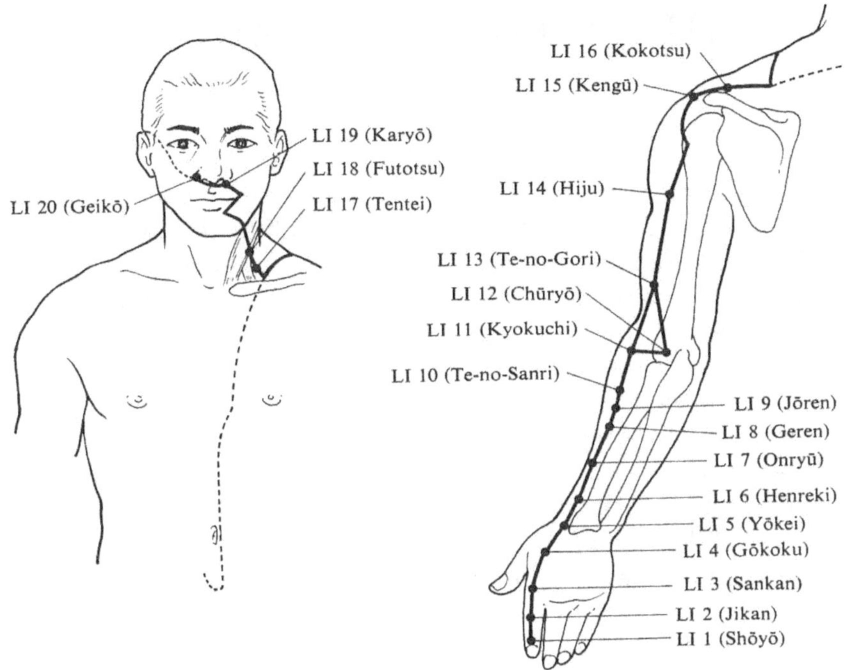

The large intestine meridian

THE STOMACH MERIDIAN

The stomach meridian begins at the comer of the nose. One branch goes to the head, while another branch enters the body and descends to the stomach. It continues down the trunk, over the front of the thigh to the outside of the knee. Continuing downward, it runs on the outside of the lower leg over the top of the foot to the second and third toes. From the top of the foot, a branch diverts to the outside comer of the first toe. Here, the spleen meridian begins.

The stomach meridian is a channel for intellectuality. It is strongly charged with heaven's force and has the effect of stabilizing, focusing, or centering intellectual activity. The stomach meridian on the right side of the body has a weak stabilizing effect, while the meridian on the left side has a strong stabilizing effect.

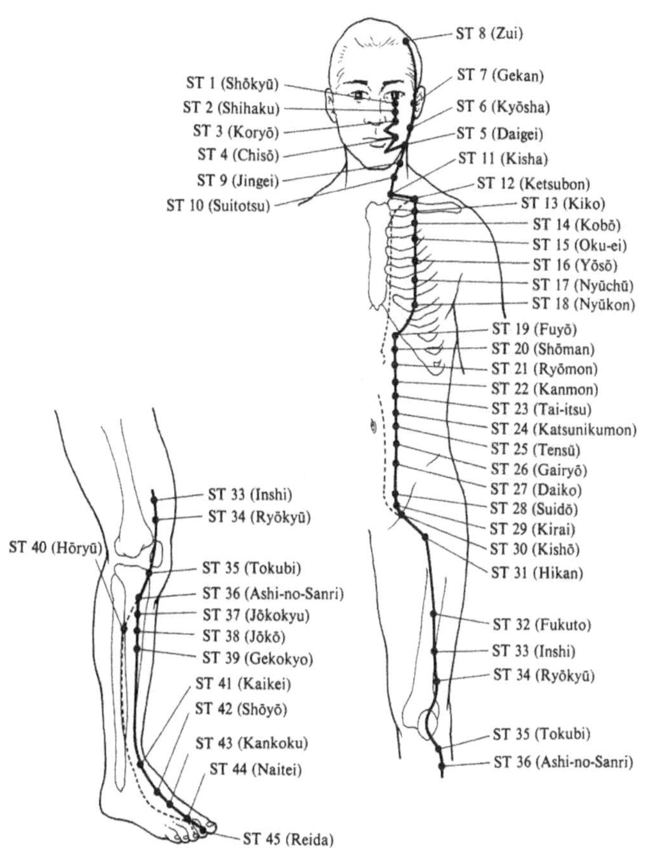

The stomach meridian

THE SPLEEN MERIDIAN

The spleen meridian begins at the outside comer of the first, or large toe, and rises along the inside of the foot above the arch around the anklebone. It ascends along the inner leg, enters the trunk and connects with the spleen. A branch of the spleen meridian goes to the three chakras in the trunk of the body, the hara chakra, the stomach chakra, and the heart chakra. A branch also ascends up the outside of the trunk and goes to the throat chakra. At the heart chakra, it connects with the heart meridian.

The spleen meridian is a channel for the emotions generated in the heart chakra, the intellectuality produced in the stomach chakra, and the social awareness originating in the hara chakra. This meridian is charged with earth's ascending energy, and therefore, activates these functions of consciousness. The spleen meridian on the right side of the body is highly charged with earth's rising power, and strongly activates these capacities. The meridian on the left side is less strongly charged by earth's energy and has a milder activating effect. Since it connects with the throat chakra, the spleen meridian also activates speech and other forms of vocal expression.

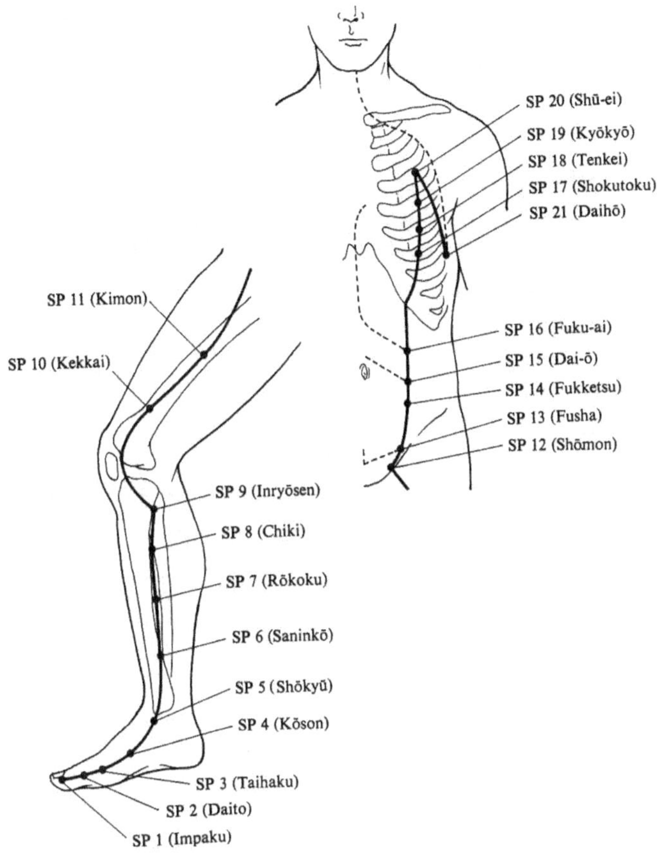

The spleen meridian

THE HEART MERIDIAN

Beginning at the heart chakra, one branch of this meridian moves upward across the chest, the side of the throat and face, to the eye. Another branch goes down to the stomach chakra and another to the armpit and down the middle of the inside of the arm to the end of the little finger on the inside. The heart meridian connects to the small intestine meridian at the end of the little finger.

The heart meridian is a channel for the emotions generated in the heart chakra and the functions of intellect originating in the stomach chakra. It is charged with earth's energy, and has an activating effect. The heart meridian on the right side strongly activates the emotions and intellect, while the meridian on the left has a weak, activating effect.

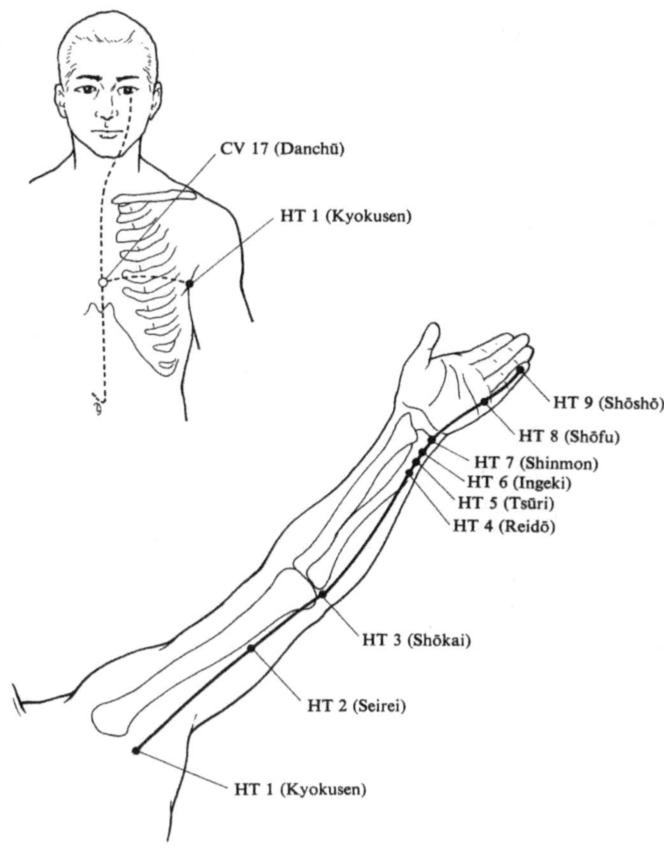

The heart meridian

THE SMALL INTESTINE MERIDIAN

The small intestine meridian begins on the outside tip of the little finger and goes back along the outside of the arm to the shoulder, where it divides into two branches. One branch goes internally down the front of the body to the small intestine, passing through the heart and stomach chakras. Another branch runs up the side of the neck to the inner comer of the eye where it connects with the bladder meridian.

The small intestine meridian acts as a channel for the emotions and intellect generated by the heart and stomach chakras. The direction of energy flow along the small intestine meridian is inward and downward, and thus it is charged primarily by heaven's yang, descending force. The small intestine meridian on the right side has a mildly inhibiting or stabilizing effect on these mental and emotional functions, while the meridian on the left side has a strong inhibiting effect.

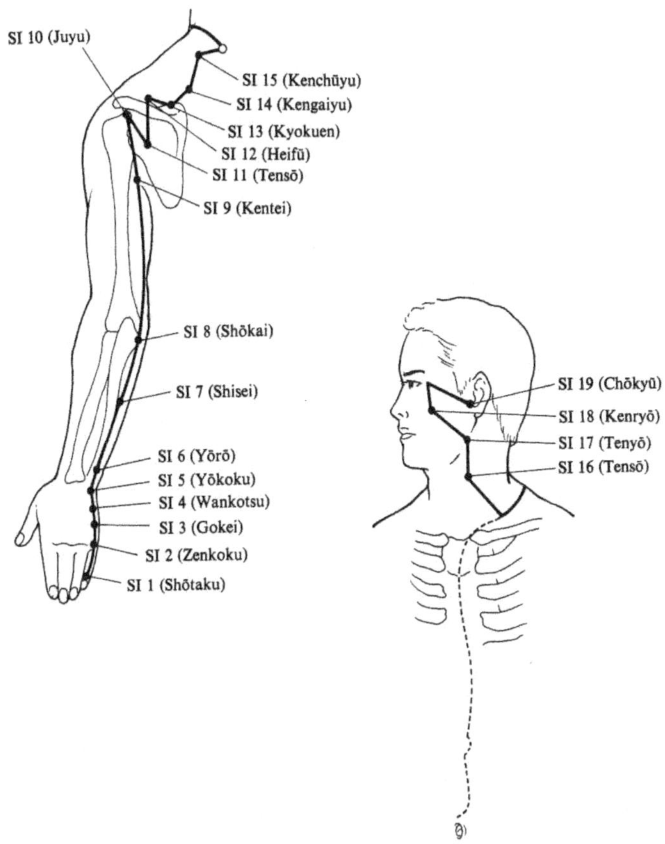

The small intestine meridian

THE BLADDER MERIDIAN

The bladder meridian begins at the inner comer of the eye and runs up across the forehead, over the head and down the neck and back. The bladder meridian connects all Yu, or entrance points on the back. At the lumbar region, a branch connects to the kidney and bladder. The meridian runs down the buttocks and the back of the legs, over the outside of the Achilles tendon, around the outside of the ankle, and over the foot to the outside of the little toe. From the little toe, it runs to the bottom of the foot where the kidney meridian begins.

The bladder meridian does not connect directly with any of the chakras. However, the Yu points on the back are connected to all the major organs, and thus the bladder meridian is indirectly linked to the throat, heart, stomach, hara, and sexual chakras. Thus the bladder meridian serves as a channel for the functions of expression, emotion, intellect, social awareness, and sexuality produced in these chakras. The bladder meridian flows downward, and is strongly charged with heaven's force. It has the effect of stabilizing or quieting these mental and emotional functions. The bladder meridian on the right side has a weak inhibiting effect; the meridian on the left has a strong inhibiting effect. Practitioners of finger pressure massage often notice that massaging down the bladder meridian can stabilize hyperactive emotions.

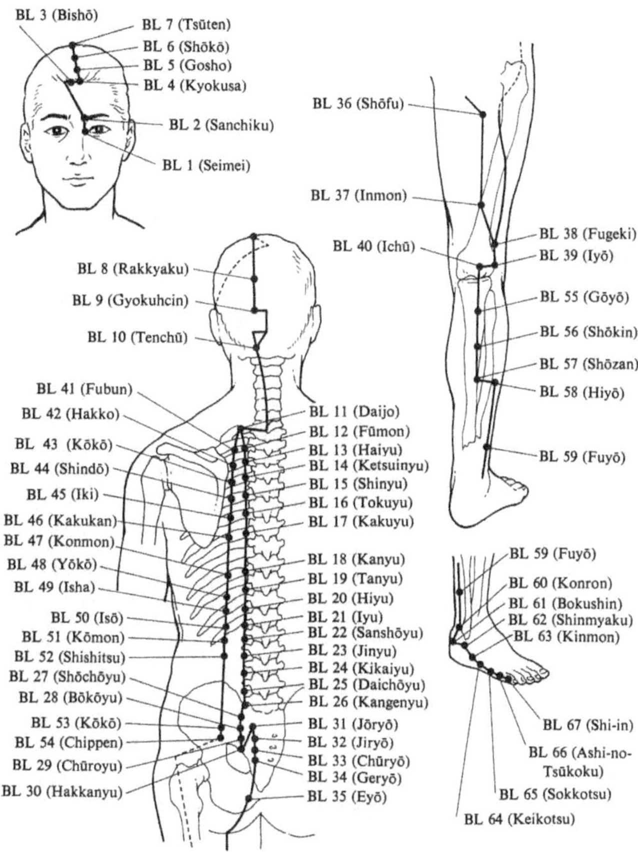

The bladder meridian

THE KIDNEY MERIDIAN

The kidney meridian begins on the sole of the foot toward the front, in the indentation between the pads formed at the base of the toes. This meridian runs along the arch of the foot, circles the inner anklebone, ascends the inside of the leg, and moves through the trunk where it connects with the sexual chakra and kidney. It then continues upward to the throat, connecting with the hara, heart, and throat chakras. A branch of the kidney meridian goes to the heart chakra where it connects to the heart governor meridian.

The kidney meridian is a channel for the functions of expression, emotion, social awareness, and sexuality generated in the chakras mentioned above. The kidney meridian flows upward and is charged by earth's expanding energy. It therefore has an activating effect on these mental and emotional functions. The kidney meridian on the right side has a strong activating effect, while the meridian on the left side has a mild activating effect.

The difference between the bladder and kidney meridians, in terms of their effects on psychological and emotional functions, can be seen in the way that massaging them affects a person's thoughts and emotions. Massaging down the bladder meridian on the back stabilizes a person's energy, calms the emotions, and deactivates sexual response. A person often becomes inwardly focused and quiet after receiving massage along the bladder meridian. Massaging up the kidney meridian on the front of the body has the opposite effect. It activates the emotions and sexual response and often causes a person to become talkative.

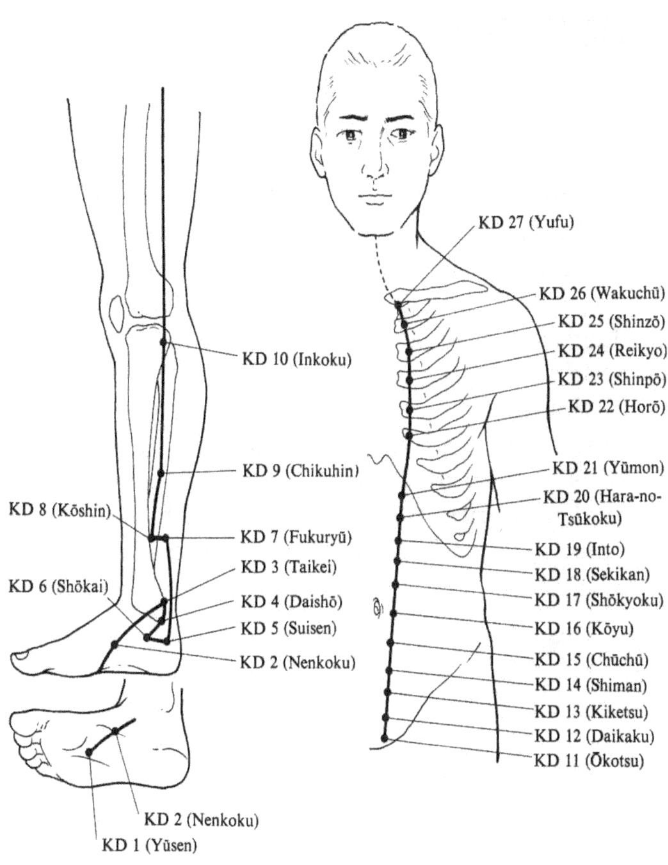

The kidney meridian

THE HEART GOVERNOR MERIDIAN

The heart governor meridian begins in the pericardium and runs across the chest and down the inside of the arm, over the center of the palm to the tip of the middle finger. A branch extends from the center of the palm to the fourth or ring finger where the triple heater meridian begins. The heart governor meridian is connected to three of the bodily chakras: the heart, stomach, and hara, and thus serves as a channel for the emotions, intellect, and social awareness generated in these chakras. The heart governor meridian is charged by earth's expanding energy and has an activating effect on these functions. The meridian on the right side has a strong activating effect; the meridian on the left side has a mild activating effect.

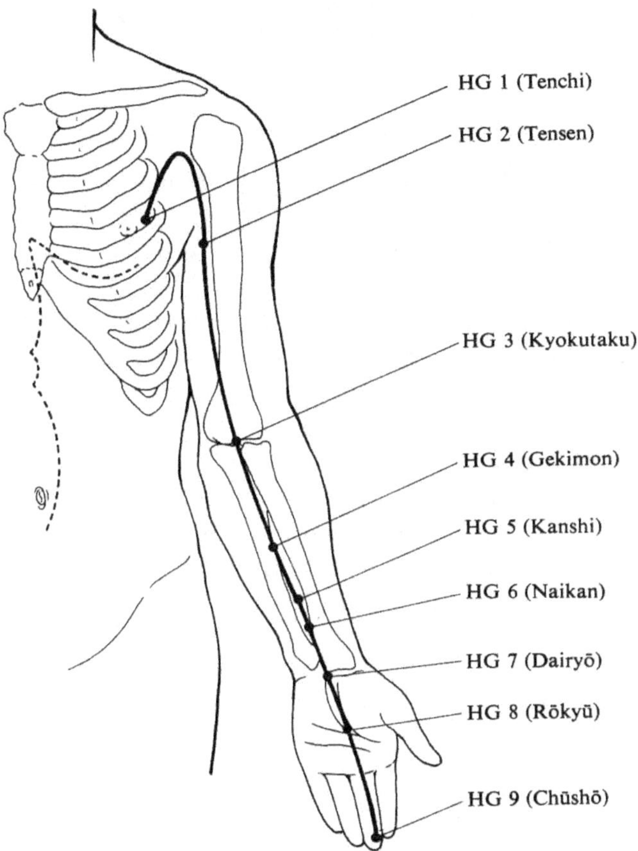

The heart governor meridian

THE TRIPLE HEATER MERIDIAN

The triple heater meridian begins at the outside of the ring finger and runs up the outside of the arm to the shoulder. One branch continues upward over the side of the head. Another branch goes to the trunk and connects the three chakras, collectively known as the triple heater—the heart, stomach, and hara chakras. The branch of the triple heater meridian that goes to the face connects with the gallbladder meridian at the end of the eyebrow.

The triple heater meridian serves as a channel for the emotional, intellectual, and social capacities generated in the heart, stomach, and hara chakras. The triple heater meridian is charged by heaven's descending energy and has a stabilizing effect on these functions. The meridian on right side has a weak stabilizing effect; the meridian on the left side has a strong stabilizing effect.

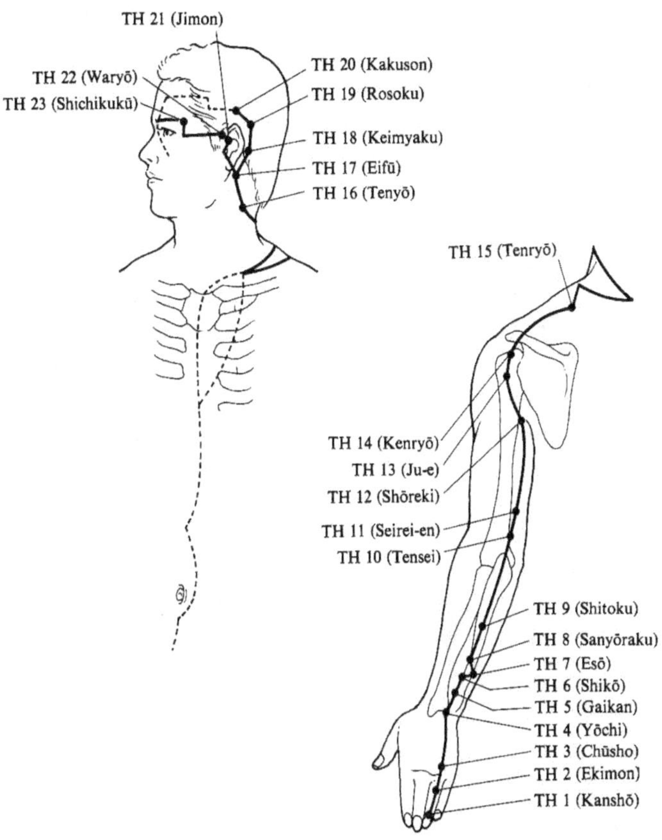

The triple heater meridian

THE GALLBLADDER MERIDIAN

One branch of the gallbladder meridian starts at the face and passes downward through the neck and chest to the gallbladder. It connects with the main branch at the hip. The main branch begins at the outside of the eyebrow and rises across the side of the head where it spirals or zigzags several times before going down the side of the neck to the top of the shoulders. It runs down the side of the trunk to the hip. From here, it goes down the outside of the leg, crossing above the anklebone, and running to the fourth toe. A branch goes to the inside of the large toe where the liver meridian begins.

The gallbladder meridian does not connect directly with the chakras. In the rib cage, it indirectly connects with the stomach chakra, and in the lower abdomen, to the sexual chakra. It thus serves as a channel for the functions of intellect and sexuality produced in these chakras. The gallbladder meridian is charged strongly with heaven's force, and thus has a stabilizing effect on these functions. The meridian on the right side of the body has a mild stabilizing effect on these functions; the meridian on the left side has a strong stabilizing effect.

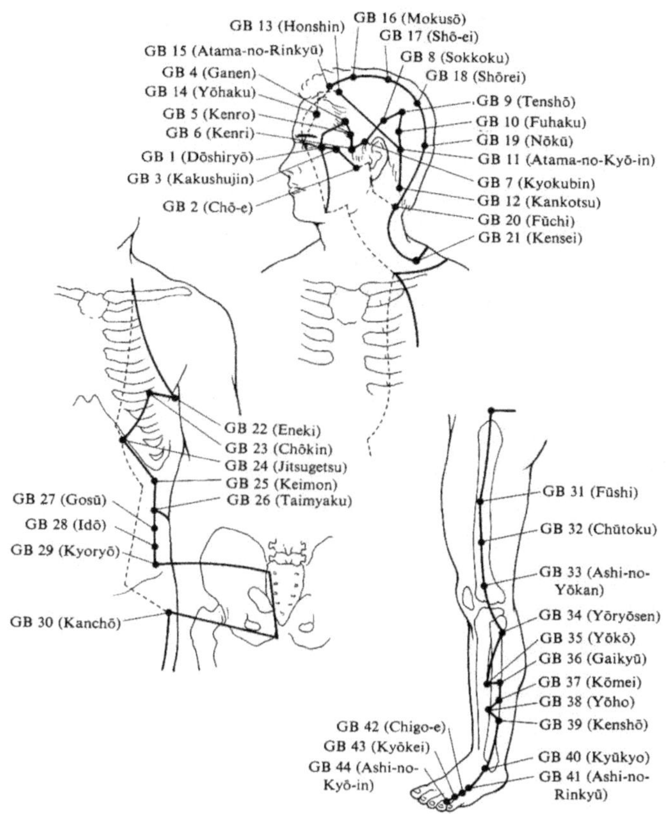

The gallbladder meridian

THE LIVER MERIDIAN

The liver meridian begins at the inside comer of the large toe and travels up the inside of the leg, enters the trunk, and moves up to the liver. This meridian continues up the trunk to the eyes, and on to the top of the head. From here, a branch goes to the stomach chakra where it connects to the first meridian, the lung meridian.

In its course through the abdomen, the liver meridian gives rise to a branch that connects with the sexual chakra. It also connects indirectly with the hara chakra, and branches into the stomach chakra. The liver meridian therefore serves as a channel for the functions of intellect, social awareness, and sexuality produced in these chakras. The liver meridian is strongly charged with earth's force, and has an activating effect on these functions. The meridian on the right side has a strong activating effect; the meridian on the left side has a milder activating effect.

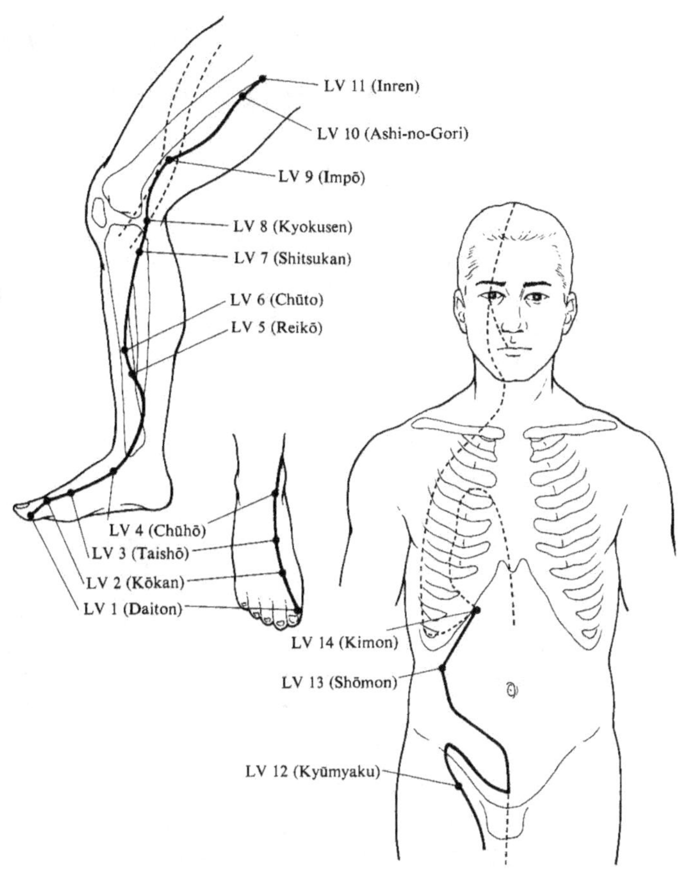

The liver meridian

THE GOVERNING & CONCEPTION VESSEL MERIDIANS

The governing vessel (GV) begins at the coccyx and flows upward on the surface of the back, along the spinal cord, over the head and down the face to the mouth. Entering the mouth, the governing vessel descends internally to the genital area, and exits at the perineum, where the cycle begins again. The governing vessel activates and strengthens our physical, mental, and spiritual abilities, together with our power to maintain the functions of life in well-coordinated harmony.

The conception vessel (CV), along with its partner, the governing vessel, constitutes the body's original meridian. Together, they form the primary channel and represent the principal flow of heaven and earth's forces within the body. Working together, they have a comprehensive influence on all physical, psychological, and spiritual functions. It is from the conception and governing vessels that the other meridians differentiate.

The conception vessel begins at the perineum, the area between the anus and genitals, and streams upward on the front surface of the body. It moves along the center of the trunk to the mouth. Entering the mouth, the conception vessel moves down the center of the body, deep inside. It exits in the area of the coccyx, the small triangular bone at the base of the spine, where it connects with the governing vessel. The conception vessel activates our spiritual, mental, and physical functions. When energy is flowing smoothly through the conception vessel, a person feels uplifted, activated, and eager to accomplish something

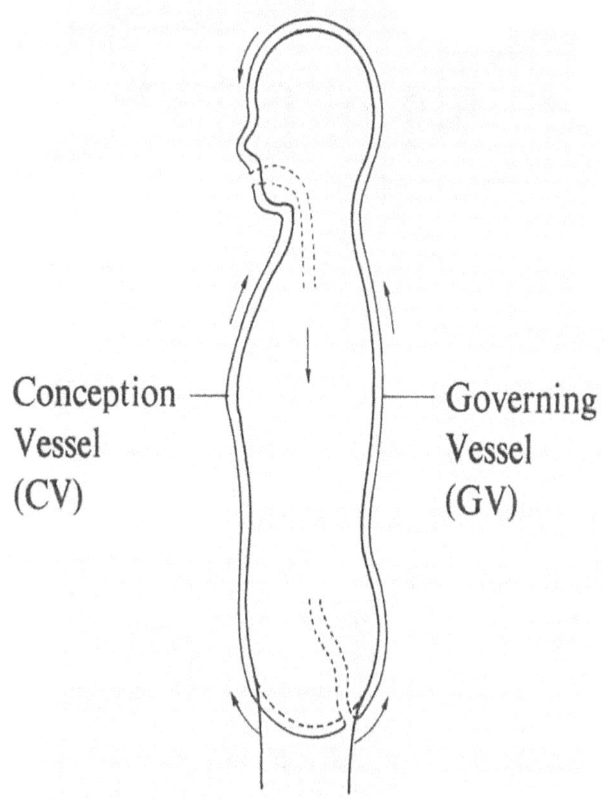

The conception vessel and governing vessel meridians

THE BODY MATRIX

The Tree of the Body is rooted in the earth and complements the invisible Tree of Consciousness. Consciousness is primarily a product of heaven's force, while the body is assembled from material substance of the earth.

On earth, the vegetable kingdom combines with elements, including air, water, and minerals, to provide the physical substance of the body. If we compare the body to clay on a potter's wheel, heaven's energy creates the motion of the wheel and acts like invisible hands that shape the clay. Heaven's force charges the entire body; it is the primary source of the life energy that streams into every cell. The body itself is composed of the material substance of the earth and is like the clay being shaped by the potter's fingers.

Like the invisible energy system, the body is formed in a way that is opposite to trees and other forms of plant life. A tree absorbs nutrients from the soil through external roots. The roots of the body are deep inside in the small intestine. It is here that nutrients are absorbed into the bloodstream and distributed to the body's cells. The branched structure of the circulatory system resembles the branched structure of a tree. It is another example of fractal division. At the most peripheral part, nutrients diffuse through minute capillaries into the cells. Cells are like the leaves of a tree. However, leaves develop externally and are open and expanded, while cells develop internally and are closed and compact.

Two complementary streams nourish each cell: one, the invisible stream of energy that enters the cell via meridian branches and the other, physical stream of nourishment entering the cell from the bloodstream.

These streams move in opposite directions: one spirals from the diffuse world of energy toward the condensed world of matter, and the other spirals from the condensed world of matter toward the world of energy.

Everyone is influenced in the same way from the universe; everyone however occupies a unique position in time and space — hence, channels heaven's energy from a different perspective. Individual differences are primarily a result of differences in the foods that people select. Food creates the unique composition of each cell. The unlimited variation in food choices creates the endless variety of physical constitutions and conditions found among people.

When a tree grows in healthy soil, it receives balanced nourishment and is able to thrive. But if the soil is deficient in minerals or contaminated with chemical toxins, the tree becomes unhealthy and its leaves eventually wither and die. A naturally balanced diet is like healthy soil. It provides the body with proper nourishment, thus ensuring sound blood and healthy functioning of each cell. If food becomes unbalanced, the blood begins to deteriorate and cells become unhealthy. The leaves of the tree depend on nutrients absorbed through the roots. Cells, including those of the brain and nervous system, depend on the nutrients passing through the small intestine. The bloodstream nourishes body and mind. By influencing the blood and cells, daily foods profoundly influence our physical health, together with our consciousness and emotions.

HEALTH OR SICKNESS

It is simple to achieve good health; it is far more difficult to make ourselves sick. To become sick, we have to eat ice cream and steak, and lead a chaotic life; otherwise, we do not become sick. It is very simple to be healthy. We need not have a chaotic life, but an ordinary, simple, modest life. Most people hate sickness. Some feel that sickness is their enemy that occurs unexpectedly and is without remedy. Others view it as stemming from misfortune or bad luck. It is difficult for them to accept that illness is something they help create.

If we yielded to changes in our environment, we would rarely become sick. However, we all have free will, or free consciousness. By exercising that free will, we go against nature, against the movement of the universe, and the result of our actions is sickness. At night we should sleep, but instead we stay awake. During the day, we should keep busy, but instead we sleep. In winter we should not take ice cream, but instead we eat a half-gallon. Our free will makes it possible for us to continuously violate nature.

If we discover the source of this freedom, we discover the secret of life and the key to health and happiness. The forces of heaven and earth flow through the body unhindered, charging and vitalizing our life functions. Heaven's force comes down and ends in the uvula. Earth's energy comes up and ends in the tongue. Between them is an open space where the forces of heaven and earth are not connected. It is here that we have a valve. By switching the valve off or on, or by opening or closing it, we decide whether these energies come in or not and whether we take in a little or a lot. We use this valve to adjust our intake in various ways, and that is how we manage our freedom. That open space is the mouth.

Our destiny is determined by the way we use our mouth. Whether we experience fortune or misfortune, health or sickness, war or peace depends entirely on it. Through breathing, we cope with the ocean of air that covers the earth. Through eating, we cope with the products of the earth itself. The energies of heaven and earth collide in the throat chakra, circulate, and are discharged in the form of organized waves known as speech. We use our eating, breathing, and speaking to manage our relationship with the environment and control our destiny. All spiritual practices eventually arrive here; for example, chanting or meditating in silence, activating or deactivating breathing, fasting, or eating in a certain way to bring forth different aspects of our spirituality.

Our thinking is also controlled in the mouth. When you think of the past, what kind of posture do you assume? Do you look downward or upward? You look downward. You bend forward and curve your body inward. Rodin's Thinker positioned downward and forward, reflects on the past. Your whole body is a spiral. In order to think of the past, you need to condense your body spiral. When you expand or relax your spiral, you are able to think of the future. When you think of the past, how do you use your mouth? Your mouth tends to be closed with your tongue attached to the palate. When you think of the future, your mouth is usually open and loose, with your tongue separated from the palate and relaxed.

In the infinite universe, beyond the world of moving phenomena, there is neither past nor future. There is only the present. In the phenomenal world, there is no present; only yin and yang, future and past. Try to hold the present. As soon as you try to grasp it, it has already become the past. Where does the present exist? The present is the infinite universe itself, which is without beginning or end and which exists beyond our relative universe. The eternal present differentiates into future and past, or yin and yang. Whether we interpret that infinite present as past or future depends on our condition. If we close our mouths and attach our tongue to the palate, we interpret these vibrations as the past. If we relax our tongue and open the mouth, we interpret them as future events.

Each of us interprets the universe based on our condition. We use our mouths differently and therefore, interpret the universe differently. As we begin to understand this, we see why people are different and, without judgment, we are able to respect these differences. We also realize that what we eat on a daily basis has a profound impact on our health.

FUTURE MEDICINE

In the future, society will embrace a new kind of medicine based on a unified view of existence. Its scope will extend well beyond modern medicine, both in the East and West. This new medicine will incorporate the most cogent points of all the world's healing systems, while modifying or completely discarding their least desirable aspects.

The new medicine will cover many areas. It will not be limited to the relief of symptoms, but will seek to change the factors that cause illness to arise, including daily food, lifestyle, and thinking. Each of these aspects is important. For example, if someone tries to eat well, yet thinks, "I can't recover, I may die," this depressed state of mind interferes with natural recovery. It is important to maintain a bright, positive outlook. Our thoughts have a direct influence on the quality of each cell. Let us now see how the macrobiotic way of life addresses these larger issues.

To help the body discharge toxins, we need to open clogged pores and sweat glands, and remove any blockage that may be impeding the flow of energy. We therefore advise scrubbing the whole body with a hot wet towel, both morning and night, and whenever possible, also removing calluses from the feet and toes. We also recommend a daily half hour walk, as it helps activate circulation and breathing; it discharges of excess and releases stagnation in both body and mind. Walking barefoot on grass, soil, or beach sand, when safe and appropriate, is helpful in charging the body with earth's electromagnetic energy.

Grounding the body in such a manner, on the earth, can help reduce pain and inflammation, strengthen the immune response, and promote deep sleep. Sing every day, preferably joyful, happy songs that uplift the spirit. Singing improves your breathing and activates energy flow.

In terms of diet, we recommend eating fewer calories, and less protein and fat. The macrobiotic diet can help everyone maintain adequate strength while developing a healthy active condition. It is not enough to limit the intake of nutrients, for example, by eating a diet of raw fruit or vegetables; for maximum health we need an adequate—but not excessive—intake of high-quality carbohydrates, protein, fats, and minerals. In order to utilize the nutrients-in whole grains, beans, vegetables, and sea vegetables, we recommend chewing well. Moreover, in order to quickly neutralize the effects of past intake of meat, eggs, cheese, poultry, milk, sugar, and other extremes, we utilize simple home remedies, including special drinks and teas made from daily foods. These simple macrobiotic remedies can be prepared at home with foods available in the kitchen.

Environmental factors are also important. The ability to discharge depends upon such factors as weather, air pressure, and humidity. In order to help the skin discharge effectively, it is better to wear clothing made of cotton and other vegetable fabrics, rather than synthetic materials and to use cotton sheets and pillowcases. In order to freshen the air in the home, it is a good idea to put green plants in the bedroom and elsewhere throughout the house. Opening the windows from time to time, even in cold weather, helps keep air circulation smooth.

Watching Netflix, playing video games, surfing the Web, talking incessantly on a cell phone, all of these activities increase radiation absorption in the body, inhibiting energy from flowing freely in the chakras and meridians. It is best to be aware of the time we spend with electromagnetic devices that to overdo it, especially when recovering from a specific health condition. When we are busy and active, this stimulates our metabolism and free flow of energy. In order to attain and maintain optimum health, it is important for us to attend to the following: the food and beverages we consume; the quality of our thinking (i.e. is it positive or negative, etc.); the environment that we interact with; and our lifestyle (which includes our daily activities.) The new medicine will address each of these key areas and treat each individual as a microcosm of the macrocosm.

Self-responsibility is another important aspect of the new medicine. After we learn to cook, eat, and orient daily life in harmony with nature, how accurately we put this knowledge into practice is entirely up to us. No one else can do such things as chew, exercise, or wear cotton clothing for us.

If we do not apply this knowledge in our lives, or if we apply it in a casual or careless manner, maintaining good health is difficult.

Therefore, we need to firmly resolve to change ourselves: to change our way of eating, thinking, and lifestyle. We must change our way of life. No one else can accomplish this for us. Everyone is entirely free; no one can control or limit this freedom. Whether we become healthy and happy, or whether we make ourselves sick and unhappy, is entirely up to us. Symptomatic medicine cannot change the cause of illness. Since we are the producers of health or sickness, we are the only ones who have the power to change our direction.

The new medicine will concentrate a large share of resources on education. It will guide people toward an understanding of humanity, and emphasize the correct way of life for everyone, including the way to develop a positive image of health and peace. The new medicine will teach everyone how to extend love and friendship to other people, and how to establish world peace.

Ultimately, the new medicine will guide humanity toward a greater spiritual awareness. Someone may believe that modem civilization, with all of its conveniences, is wonderful, and that foods such as steak and hamburger are desirable as symbols of material success. In order to realize health, however, we must change this view of life to one that is more harmonious with nature. Our whole way of life must change. We must shift away from egocentric thinking toward a universal understanding. We need to realize that we are a part of nature and that we have to adapt and change with it rather than exploit it for selfish purposes. Self-reflection can lead everyone toward a humble and modest way of life, a way of life filled with love and gratitude.

The medicine of the future will help solve the problems of human existence. It will utilize simple, natural methods to treat the symptoms of disease, and will be based on a clear understanding of the psychological and spiritual causes of illness. It will guide everyone toward a way of life in harmony with nature and the universe. As a true biological and spiritual change take place, humanity will become a more elevated species.

Modem intellectual humanity—Homo sapiens—will evolve into a new species, *Homo spiritus*. This new species will live in harmony with each other and with their environment on earth, and will see the end of war, crime, violence, and degenerative disease.

They will naturally share a sense of brother and sisterhood, and establish an enduring peace. The new medicine will thus lead humanity away from sickness toward planetary health and peace. It will open the door to a new world.

Resources

International Macrobiotic Institute, PO Box 2051, Lenox, MA 01240. Sponsor of the Macrobiotic Online Course and the Nine Star Ki Online Course. Publisher of IMI Press titles. Visit InternationalMacrobioticInstitute.com for information.

Planetary Health/Amberwaves, PO Box 487, Becket MA 01223, 413-623-0012, email: shenwa@bcn.net, www.amberwaves.org. Sponsor of the Macrobiotic Summer Conference and the Online Macrobiotic Winter Conference. Publisher of various books and periodicals. Visit MacrobioticSummerConference.com. A 501(c)(3) non-profit organization.

Macrobiotics Today/George Ohsawa Macrobiotic Foundation (GOMF), 1277 Marian Ave., Chico CA 95928, 800-232-2372, gomf@OhsawaMacrobiotics.com, www.OhsawaMacrobiotics.com. Publisher of *Macrobiotics Today*.

About Michio Kushi

Michio Kushi, a leading figure in the macrobiotic movement, began his study of macrobiotics more than sixty years ago and went on to establish the Kushi Institute in Massachusetts. As the leading voice in the macrobiotic community, he was the best-selling author of over twenty books on the macrobiotic lifestyle, including *The Book of Macrobiotics, Macrobiotic Home Remedies,* and *Your Body Never Lies. —* **From *One Peaceful World.***

The Macrobiotic Online Course

In this first of its kind course combining video, audio, print, and live interaction, students have the opportunity to study all facets of macrobiotics with Edward Esko, longtime associate of Michio Kushi and Founder of the International Macrobiotic Institute (IMI). The Macrobiotic Online Course is designed to enable students to gain ongoing benefit from their practice of macrobiotics while helping develop the skills needed to guide and counsel others. For details go to InternationalMacrobioticInstitute.com.